Is It Heartburn Or HeartAttack?

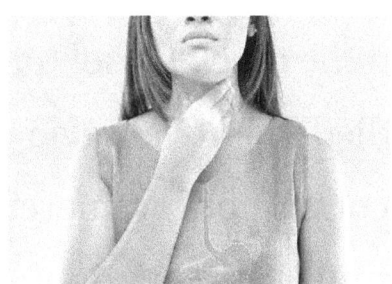

Know The Difference Between Heartburn And HeartAttack

Martha J. Jones

All may be reproduced, distributed, or transmitted in any form or by any means, including photocopying, recording, or other electronic or mechanical methods, without the prior written permission of the publisher, except in the case of brief quotations embodied in critical reviews and certain other noncommercial uses permitted by copyright law.

Copyright © Martha J. Jones, 2022.

Table of contents
Chapter 1
Chapter 2

Chapter 1
What is Heartburn?

Heartburn is a searing discomfort in your chest, directly beneath your breastbone. Heartburn is a burning sensation in the chest produced by stomach acid going up into the esophagus (acid reflux). If it continues occurring, it's termed gastro-oesophageal reflux disease (GORD). Occasional heartburn is frequent and has no reason for panic. Most individuals may manage the pain of heartburn on their own with lifestyle modifications and nonprescription drugs. Heartburn that is more frequent or interferes with your everyday routine may be an indication of a more severe problem that needs medical attention.

The American College of Gastroenterology estimates that more than 15 million individuals in the United States have heartburn symptoms every day.

Heartburn is more likely during pregnancy. Most individuals develop heartburn after meals, but may also awaken people when they are asleep. People also may develop heartburn after eating particular meals or drinking certain drinks

How long does heartburn last?

Heartburn may affect individuals differently. In general, heartburn symptoms begin immediately after eating and may continue anywhere from a few minutes to a couple of hours, or even longer.

How long you endure symptoms depends on the underlying reason. It also relies on what you do at the first indication of symptoms. For example, sometimes heartburn sensations continue until your body digests the triggering meal. Other times, the discomfort goes away if you stand up instead of reclining down after eating.

If you use over the counter (OTC) antacids or prescription drugs as part of a treatment plan, you may have a shorter duration or fewer heartburn symptoms.

SYMPTOMS OF HEARTBURN

Chest discomfort may be an indication of a heart attack. Seek attention immediately away if you experience significant chest discomfort or pressure, particularly when paired with pain in the arm or jaw or trouble breathing.

Make an appointment with your health care practitioner if:

- heartburn — a burning feeling in the center of your chest. Heartburn happens more than twice a week
- You have difficulties swallowing
- You experience recurrent nausea or vomiting
- You suffer weight loss because of reduced appetite or difficulties eating
- An unpleasant sour sensation in your mouth, produced by stomach acid
- A cough or hiccups that keep coming again
- A hoarse voice
- Bad breath
- Bloating and feeling unwell

- Symptoms persist despite the usage of nonprescription drugs.

Symptoms are generally worse after eating, while laying down and when leaning over.

How Heartburn And GERD Occur?

Heartburn happens when stomach acid backs up into the tube that delivers food from your mouth to your stomach (esophagus).

The esophagus is a tube that links the mouth to the stomach. It is formed of muscles that operate to push food into the stomach in periodic waves. Once in the stomach, food is blocked from refluxing (going back into the esophagus), by a specific section of circular muscle positioned at the junction of the esophagus and stomach, termed the lower esophageal sphincter (LES).

A pressure differential across the diaphragm, the flat muscle that divides the chest from the belly, also tends to retain stomach contents in the stomach.
The stomach puts food, acids, and enzymes together to begin digestion. There are specific protective cells that coat the stomach to prevent the acid from creating irritation. The esophagus does not have this same protection, and if stomach acid and digestive fluids reflux back into the esophagus, they may cause irritation and damage to its vulnerable lining.

Typically, when food is eaten, a ring of muscle surrounding the bottom of the esophagus (lower esophageal sphincter) relaxes to enable food and fluids to pass down into the stomach. Then the muscle tightens again.

If the lower esophageal sphincter isn't acting as it should, stomach acid may flow back up into the esophagus (acid reflux) and produce heartburn. The acid backup may be worse while you're bent over or laying down.

Causes of heartburn

Lots of individuals have heartburn from time to time. There's frequently no evident explanation why.

Sometimes it's caused or made worse by:
- ☐ Spicy foods
- ☐ Being overweight
- ☐ Smoking

- ☐ Pregnancy
- ☐ Stress and anxiety
- ☐ Citrus products
- ☐ Tomato products, such as ketchup
- ☐ Fatty or fried meals
- ☐ Peppermint
- ☐ Chocolate
- ☐ Alcohol, carbonated beverages, coffee, or other caffeinated drinks
- ☐ Large or fatty meals
- ☐ A rise in certain kinds of hormones, such as progesterone and oestrogen
- ☐ Various drugs, such as anti-inflammatory painkillers (like ibuprofen).
- ☐ A hiatus hernia — when part of your stomach rises into your chest.

Complications

Heartburn is not without consequences. If untreated, recurring irritation and inflammation of the esophagus may develop into ulcers, which are tiny pockets of tissue disintegration. These may cause significant bleeding.

Heartburn that happens regularly and interferes with a daily routine is labeled gastroesophageal reflux disease (GERD). GERD treatment may require prescription medications and, occasionally, surgery or other procedures. GERD may badly damage your esophagus or develop into precancerous alterations in the esophagus called Barrett's esophagus. Other concerns include food pipe inflammation and a variety of breathing difficulties that might include: asthma, fluid in the lungs, coughing, a sore throat, hoarseness, pneumonia wheezing.

Heartburn Diagnosis

Heartburn is a frequent complaint, yet it may be mistaken for other chest-related ailments, including heart attack, pulmonary embolus, pneumonia, and chest wall discomfort.

The diagnosis starts with a full history and physical examination. In many circumstances, those offer enough information for the health care practitioner to establish the diagnosis and initiate a treatment plan. In certain circumstances, extra testing may be required:

X-ray: The patient may be asked to drink barium or Gastrografin (two kinds of contrast materials) while a radiologist, using an X-ray or fluoroscopy system, observes the contrast material traveling down the esophagus and entering into the stomach. Aside from looking for irregularities or inflammation within the esophagus and of the esophageal walls, this test can determine if the esophagus muscles are working properly in a rhythmic fashion to push the contrast material into the stomach.

Endoscopy: In this examination, a gastroenterologist uses a flexible scope and a fiber optic camera to look at the lining of the esophagus and stomach. Inflammation and ulcers may be recognized. Biopsies and tiny fragments of tissue may be collected to search for malignant or pre-cancerous cells.

Manometry and pH testing: Less often, when conventional treatment has failed to confirm the diagnosis, or when symptoms are unusual, the use of pressure monitors and acid measures from inside the esophagus may be useful in determining the diagnosis.

Ambulatory acid (pH) probe test. Your doctor will pass a small tube through your nose into your esophagus. A sensor at the tip of the tube measures the amount of stomach acid in your esophagus.

Esophageal pH monitoring. Your doctor puts a capsule on the lining of your esophagus to assess acid reflux.

Remedies

Using basic lifestyle and behavioral strategies may help avoid or lessen heartburn. Suggestions include:
- ☐ Following a balanced diet, with a minimal fat intake.
- ☐ Avoid eating 2–3 hours before night. Eat meals at least three to four hours before you lay down. This allows your stomach time to empty and minimizes the possibility of getting heartburn overnight.

- ☐ Raising the head of the bed before sleeping down.
- ☐ Avoid wearing tight-fitting garments, Wear loose-fitting clothes to reduce unwanted strain on the tummy.
- ☐ Avoiding excessive lifting and straining to avoid eating triggers, such as alcohol, coffee, spicy food, acidic meals, or foods producing gas and bloating.
- ☐ Acquiring or maintaining a modest weight.
- ☐ Stop smoking, if appropriate, and prevent secondhand smoke.
- ☐ Exercising regularly, eating smaller meals more often.
- ☐ Avoid overeating. Cutting down on the number of your servings during meals

will help minimize your risk of heartburn. You might also try eating four or five little meals instead of three bigger ones.

☐ Slowing down. Eating slowly may frequently help avoid heartburn. Put your fork down between bites and avoid eating too hastily.

☐ Avoiding certain meals. For many individuals, particular meals aggravate heartburn. Avoiding these meals may help. Try maintaining track of these meals so that you can look out for them in the future. Your healthcare practitioner may also urge that you avoid alcohol.

☐ Consider prescription medications: People with heartburn should also discuss with their doctor the usage of prescription drugs and if they are good for the individual.

☐ Manage body weight: People who are overweight or obese may discover that lowering body weight may assist. A diet and exercise weight-loss program may assist to minimize symptoms of acid reflux.

It is of note, however, that these lifestyle alterations may not work for everyone.

Possible Treatment:(Medications)

- Antacids.

These drugs help neutralize gastric acid. They may give fast alleviation of heartburn symptoms. Common antacids are:

Mylanta

Rolaids

Tums

Alka-Seltzer

Gaviscon

How do antacids work to relieve heartburn? Antacids help neutralize the acid your stomach generates. They give quick, short-term alleviation of heartburn symptoms. Antacids act differently from H2 blockers and PPIs, which lower or block stomach acid.

They are not meant for everyday use. You should take antacids shortly after eating or when you experience symptoms.

Antacids come in liquid, tablet, or gummy form. Most contain one or more of the following ingredients:

calcium

Aluminum

magnesium

Antacids are normally regarded as safe, however, they may induce certain adverse effects, such as diarrhea or constipation. Make careful to follow the advice on the package and avoid overusing antacids. Talk with your doctor if you have any concerns about using an antacid or if you suffer any issues after taking one.

- Histamine-2 (H2) blockers.

H2 blockers lower the amount of acid your stomach generates. They include:

Cimetidine (Tagamet HB)
Famotidine (Pepcid Complete or Pepcid AC)
Nizatidine (Axid AR)
Proton pump inhibitors (PPIs). PPIs lessen the quantity of acid in your stomach. They may also help mend damaged tissue in your esophagus.

They include:
Lansoprazole (Prevacid 24 HR)
Esomeprazole (Nexium 24 HR)
Omeprazole magnesium (Prilosec)
Omeprazole with sodium bicarbonate (Zegerid).

Although some drugs may be useful, they may have negative effects, according to the NIDDKTrusted Source. Antacids may produce constipation or diarrhea. PPIs may induce headaches, diarrhea, or upset stomach. Talk with your doctor about any drugs you're already taking to determine whether you're at risk for any drug interactions.

If over-the-counter (OTC) drugs do not help your symptoms, your doctor may be able to prescribe stronger versions of these treatments.

Chapter 2

Heartburn During Pregnancy

According to the Office on Women's Health (OWH)Trusted Source, heartburn, and indigestion are normal in pregnancy owing to hormonal changes and the baby pushing on the stomach.

The OWH advises certain food and lifestyle adjustments that may help ease the symptoms. These include:

Eating five to six small meals throughout the day.

Not laying down within an hour after eating avoiding fatty and spicy foods.

What Causes Heartburn During Pregnancy?

Causes of heartburn during pregnancy include:

Hormone Levels Changing: Your hormone levels vary throughout pregnancy, impacting how you accept and digest meals. The hormones often slow down your digestive system. Food goes slowly, producing bloating and heartburn.

Esophageal Sphincter Relaxing: Progesterone, known as the pregnancy hormone, may induce the lower esophageal sphincter to relax. When it relaxes, stomach acid might travel up into the esophagus.

Uterus Enlarging: As your baby develops, your uterus becomes larger. It may compress your stomach and drive stomach acids upward, entering your esophagus. That's why heartburn is more frequent during the third trimester, the final few months of pregnancy. The baby and uterus are largest then, overwhelming your other organs.

Heartburn Or Heart Attack?

A heart attack occurs when the arteries linked to the heart get clogged. Heartburn, on the other hand, happens when stomach acid flows back up the esophagus.

Some symptoms of heartburn and a heart attack might be identical, such as chest discomfort. As a consequence, some individuals who are suffering from a heart attack do not take action as they assume they have heartburn.

If a person suffers heartburn discomfort with shortness of breath or sweating, this might indicate a heart-related condition. Other signs of a heart attack might include:

discomfort in the chest, such as squeezing, fullness, pressure, or pain
nausea
lightheadedness
pain or discomfort in one or both arms, stomach, neck, jaw, or back.

Warning indications of a heart attack generally involve discomfort in the chest that extends to the shoulders, neck, or arms. The individual may acquire a cold sweat, dizziness, shortness of breath, and potentially nausea and vomiting. These symptoms seldom or rarely occur with heartburn.

If a person experiences any or all of these symptoms, they should seek immediate medical assistance. In the words of the

American Heart Association (AHA), "If in doubt, check it out."

Knowing how to identify a heart attack from heartburn may save lives.

Foods That Help Prevent Heartburn (Acid Reflux)

There are many things you can consume to help avoid acid reflux. Stock your kitchen with goods from these three categories:

- A bowl of banana oatmeal
- High-fiber foods

Fibrous foods make you feel full so you're less likely to overeat, which may contribute to heartburn. So, load up on healthy fiber from these foods:

Whole grains such as oatmeal, couscous, and brown rice.

Root vegetables such as sweet potatoes, carrots, and beets.

Green vegetables such as asparagus, broccoli, and green beans.

A bowl of mixed nuts

- Alkaline foods

Foods fall somewhere along the pH scale (an indicator of acid levels) (an indicator of acid levels). Those that have a low pH are acidic and more likely to cause reflux. Those with higher pH are alkaline and may help balance severe stomach acid. Alkaline foods include:

Bananas

Melons

Cauliflower

Fennel

Nuts

A dish of sliced watermelon

- Watery meals

Eating meals that contain a lot of water might dilute and decrease gastric acid. Choose foods such as:

Celery

Cucumber

Lettuce

Watermelon

Broth-based soups

Herbal tea

WILL WATER EASE YOUR GERD SYMPTOMS?

Our bodies are between 55 and 60% water. When you don't drink enough to be adequately hydrated, you might have headaches, dry mouth, tiredness, and lack of attention. Not having enough to drink may also hamper regular digestion, which can lead to constipation and poor nutrition. But, water needs to be drunk at the appropriate moments to aid with GERD symptoms.

Sometimes, when heartburn symptoms begin, a few sips of water can offer relief. This might be the consequence of water-neutralizing acids and washing them out of the esophagus. Water has a pH that, at 7, is neutral. This dilutes the more acidic stomach juices, offering comfort.

But when you have eaten a meal that is too big, drinking water at the same time or quickly after might make GERD symptoms worse. Be careful about overeating and drink water gently with a meal instead of gulping down big portions. Too much volume may make the stomach bloated, resulting in increased pressure on the lower esophageal sphincter.

Drinking water during the latter stages of digestion helps lessen acidity and GERD symptoms. Often, there are pockets of high acidity, between a pH of 1 and 2, immediately below the esophagus. By consuming tap or filtered water a short time after a meal, you may dilute the acid there, which can result in reduced heartburn.

In general, you can best reduce GERD symptoms by drinking little quantities with your meal; just enough to make eating pleasant. Save bigger glasses for between meals to keep you well-hydrated and healthy.

www.ingramcontent.com/pod-product-compliance
Lightning Source LLC
Chambersburg PA
CBHW050325220526
45465CB00005B/2135